Blood Type Nutrition and Exercise

How to Use Your Blood Type to Optimize Your Diet and Fitness Routine

Betty B. Burton

Table of Contents

Introduction

In a world inundated with generic health advice, where one-size-fits-all solutions dominate the shelves, have you ever felt lost in the crowd, wondering why that diet or exercise plan just doesn't seem to work for you? What if the key to unlocking your ultimate health and fitness isn't a trendy fad or a universal regimen, but something as unique and intrinsic as your blood?

Welcome to "Blood Type Nutrition and Exercise: How to Use Your Blood Type to Optimize Your Diet and Fitness Routine." This book is not just another health guide; it's a revelation, a tailored roadmap to your well-being based on the incredible, often overlooked power of your blood type.

Have you ever wondered why some people thrive on a high-protein diet while others seem to glow with plant-based meals? Or why do certain fitness routines yield remarkable results for some but leave others drained and disheartened? The secret lies within the very essence that courses through your veins, your blood type.

Prepare to embark on a journey that unveils the profound connection between your blood type and the food you eat, the exercises you do, and the lifestyle choices you make. Imagine discovering a way of eating and moving that feels effortless, effective, and above all uniquely yours.

This book isn't just about what to eat or how to exercise; it's about a personal transformation, a revelation that can change the way you perceive health and fitness forever. Join me as we explore the untapped potential of your blood type and unlock the doors to your optimum health and vitality.

Get ready to rewrite the rules and reclaim your health in a way that's deeply, authentically you. Because, in the end, true wellness isn't about conforming to a trend; it's about honoring the incredible blueprint you carry within you, your blood.

Are you ready to unleash the power of your blood type and sculpt a lifestyle that resonates with your very core? It's time to redefine what it means to be truly, uniquely healthy.

Chapter 1

Blood Type Basics

Exploring the Different Blood Types

In a world striving for universality, it's incredibly refreshing to discover that our individuality extends to our very blood. Each of us falls into one of four blood types, Type O, Type A, Type B, or Type AB. These blood types are not just biological labels; they are a gateway to understanding your body and achieving a level of health and wellness that feels truly personalized.

The DNA of Blood Types

Blood types are determined by specific proteins found on the surface of red blood cells. The two main blood group systems that we commonly refer to are the ABO system (with Types A, B, AB, and O) and the Rh system (positive or negative). These blood groups are a result of the genes passed down from our parents, and they play a pivotal role in how our bodies function.

Understanding your blood type is like discovering the secret code to your body's preferences, strengths, and vulnerabilities. It's your unique user manual for a healthier, happier life.

The Key Players: Type O, Type A, Type B, and Type AB

Type O: The Omnivores

Type O individuals, often called the "universal donors," have a robust and adaptable metabolism. They thrive on high-protein diets and are known for their strength and resilience. In this section, we'll delve into what makes Type O special, what they should eat, and how they can best exercise to unlock their full potential.

Type A: The Agrarians

Type A individuals, on the other hand, have a more sensitive digestive system. Their bodies lean towards plant-based nutrition, and they often find peace through gentler, holistic exercise. We'll explore the characteristics that define Type A, what their ideal diet looks like, and how they can embrace their uniqueness to achieve optimal well-being.

Type B: The Nomads

Type B individuals have a fascinating balance between Type O and Type A. They can handle a variety of foods and exercise regimens. Discover the strengths of Type B, what fuels their bodies best, and how they can harness their innate potential.

Type AB: The Enigmas

Type AB is the rarest of the blood types and combines traits from both Type A and Type B. These individuals are adaptable and versatile. We'll unravel the enigma that is Type AB, exploring their dietary and exercise needs to support their complex biology.

Why This Matters

Understanding your blood type isn't just about categorization; it's about empowerment. It's about crafting a lifestyle that aligns with your unique genetic blueprint, one that offers sustainable health benefits and real results. It's not a fad; it's a shift towards authenticity, positivity, and an improved quality of life.

By the end of this chapter, you'll gain the insights you need to identify your blood type and begin tailoring your nutrition and exercise routines accordingly. It's a journey towards a more vital, healthier, and happier you, one that's firmly rooted in your individuality.

So, let's embark on this enlightening journey of self-discovery and harness the power of your blood type to optimize your diet and fitness routine. The path to a healthier, more vibrant you awaits, and it begins right here, with your unique blood type.

Genetic Implications and Health Associations

Our blood type is not just a random label; it's an intricate part of our genetic makeup that holds profound implications for our health. In this section, we'll explore the fascinating world of genetic implications and health associations related to blood types. By understanding these connections, you'll gain valuable insights into how your blood type can impact your overall well-being.

The Genetic Basis of Blood Types

At the core of our blood types are specific genes that we inherit from our parents. The ABO blood group system, which categorizes individuals into Types A, B, AB, and O, is determined by the presence or absence of antigens on the surface of red blood cells. These antigens are inherited through a combination of genetic markers passed down from our ancestors.

Type A: Individuals with Type A blood have A antigens on their red blood cells, and they carry the A gene.

Type B: Type B individuals have B antigens and carry the B gene.

Type AB: This group has both A and B antigens, indicating the presence of both A and B genes.

Type O: Type O individuals lack A and B antigens, possessing neither the A nor the B gene.

The Rh factor, another key component, determines whether an individual is Rh-positive (+) or Rh-negative (-). This factor is inherited independently from the ABO blood group, resulting in eight possible blood types.

Health Associations

Disease Susceptibility

Different blood types are associated with varying susceptibility to certain diseases and health conditions. These associations provide valuable insights for personalized health management.

Type O: Type O individuals are believed to have a lower risk of heart disease but may be more susceptible to certain infections. Their robust immune system is thought to be responsible for this lower risk of heart disease.

Type A: Type A individuals may have a higher risk of heart disease, but they tend to fare better with vegetarian and plant-based diets. They may also be more susceptible to stress-related health issues.

Type B: Type B individuals are thought to have a lower risk of heart disease compared to Type A, but they might be more susceptible to autoimmune diseases. Their ability to adapt to various diets is a notable characteristic.

Type AB: Type AB individuals often possess a mix of Type A and Type B traits. While they may have some advantages, they might also be more prone to certain conditions. Their diet and lifestyle should aim to strike a balance between Type A and Type B recommendations.

Blood Clotting and Blood Type
Blood clotting tendencies can vary based on blood type. Type O individuals tend to have a lower risk of blood clot formation, while Type A individuals might be more susceptible to clot-related conditions.

Pregnancy and Blood Type
A pregnant woman's blood type can affect her baby's health. Rh incompatibility can lead to complications during pregnancy and childbirth, highlighting the importance of

understanding blood type in family planning and prenatal care.

Blood Type and Nutrition

Blood type can influence how our bodies digest and process different foods. It's not just about dietary preferences; it's about optimizing your nutrition to support your genetic makeup.

By understanding the genetic implications and health associations related to your blood type, you can make more informed choices about your diet, exercise routine, and overall lifestyle. It's a path toward personalized wellness, where you can harness the power of your genetics to achieve better health and vitality. In the following chapters, we'll explore how to apply this knowledge practically to create a healthier and more vibrant you.

Chapter 2

Blood Type and Diet

Type O: The Omnivores

In this chapter, we embark on a journey to discover the dietary preferences and health considerations for Type O individuals, often referred to as "The Omnivores" of the blood type. If you're a Type O, you're in for a fascinating exploration of how your blood type influences your nutritional needs, offering you a roadmap to better health, vitality, and well-being.

Type O Characteristics

Type O individuals are often characterized as the earliest blood type, tracing their ancestry back to the hunter-gatherer era. They are hailed as the "Omnivores" for their ability to adapt to a wide range of foods. Here's a glimpse into what defines Type O:

Strength and Resilience: Type O individuals are known for their robust physicality and natural strength.

Historically, they were the hunters and gatherers who thrived on intense physical activity.

High Acid Levels: Type O individuals tend to have higher stomach acid levels, which aid in digesting animal proteins efficiently. This makes them well-suited to a meat-based diet.

Greater Tolerance for Fats: Their bodies are more tolerant of fats, which means they can incorporate healthy fats into their diets.

Susceptibility to Digestive Issues: On the flip side, Type O individuals might be more prone to digestive issues and food sensitivities, particularly when they consume gluten or dairy products.

The Type O Diet

The Type O diet is designed to complement their genetic makeup, enhance their strengths, and address their vulnerabilities. Here's an overview of dietary recommendations for Type O individuals:

Lean Protein: Protein from animal sources, such as lean meat, poultry, and fish, is essential for Type-O individuals. They can thrive on a high-protein diet.

Avoid Dairy: Lactose, the sugar found in dairy, can be challenging for Type O individuals to digest. They are often advised to limit or avoid dairy products.

Limit Grains: Grains, especially those containing gluten, can be problematic for Type O individuals. It's recommended to reduce or eliminate wheat and other gluten-containing grains.

Embrace Vegetables: Non-starchy vegetables, such as leafy greens, broccoli, and sweet potatoes, are beneficial for Type O individuals. These provide essential nutrients and fiber.

Moderate Fruit: Type O individuals can enjoy a variety of fruits, but they should be mindful of portion sizes and choose less acidic fruits.

Healthy Fats: Incorporate healthy fats, such as olive oil and nuts, into the diet. These fats support overall health.

Meal Planning for Type O

Creating balanced, satisfying meals for Type O individuals involves careful consideration of the recommended food groups. Here's an example of a Type O meal plan:

Breakfast: Scrambled eggs with spinach and a side of berries.

Lunch: Grilled chicken salad with mixed greens, avocado, and vinaigrette dressing.

Snack: A handful of mixed nuts.

Dinner: Baked salmon with steamed broccoli and quinoa.

Achieving Optimal Health

The Type O diet isn't just about what you should eat; it's about optimizing your health and well-being. By aligning your nutrition with your blood type, you can harness your innate strengths, mitigate potential weaknesses, and experience increased energy, improved digestion, and enhanced overall vitality.

As you continue on this journey of self-discovery, remember that you are unique, and your dietary needs should be, too. Embrace your Type O status as an opportunity to make informed, positive changes in your life, and stay motivated to achieve your health and wellness goals. The path to a healthier and more vibrant you start with understanding your blood type and making choices that honor your genetic heritage.

Type A: The Agrarians

In this section, we delve into the fascinating world of Type A individuals, often referred to as "The Agrarians" of the blood types. If you're a Type A, you're about to embark on a journey of discovery, a journey that will shed light on how your blood type can shape your dietary preferences and health, offering you a personalized roadmap to greater well-being.

Type A Characteristics

Type A individuals are thought to have evolved as farming and agriculture became more prominent in human history. As the "Agrarians," they possess certain characteristics that make them unique:

Sensitivity: Type A individuals tend to have a more sensitive immune system and digestive tract. They may be prone to allergies and food sensitivities.

Lower Stomach Acid: They typically have lower stomach acid levels compared to Type O individuals, which can affect their ability to digest animal proteins.

Stress Sensitivity: Type A individuals often have a heightened response to stress, which can impact their overall health.

Adaptation to Vegetarian Diets: Their bodies tend to thrive on plant-based diets, making them more inclined toward vegetarianism.

The Type A Diet
The Type A diet is designed to complement their genetic makeup, focusing on foods that support their overall health and well-being. Here are some key dietary recommendations for Type A individuals:

Plant-Based Diet: Type A individuals should emphasize plant-based foods like vegetables, fruits, legumes, and whole grains. These foods provide essential nutrients and fiber.

Lean Proteins: While they may choose to include some animal proteins, lean poultry and fish are preferred over red meat. They should consume animal products in moderation.

Avoid Dairy: Dairy products, especially those high in saturated fats, are typically not well-tolerated by Type A individuals. Plant-based milk alternatives are a better choice.

Gluten Sensitivity: Type A individuals are more prone to gluten sensitivity. They should opt for gluten-free grains like quinoa, rice, and millet.

Mindful Eating: Due to their stress sensitivity, Type A individuals benefit from mindful eating practices. Stress reduction techniques and relaxation are essential parts of their lifestyle.

Meal Planning for Type A

Creating balanced, satisfying meals for Type A individuals involves thoughtful consideration of the recommended food groups. Here's an example of a Type A meal plan:

Breakfast: Oatmeal topped with fresh berries and almond butter.

Lunch: Quinoa and vegetable stir-fry with tofu.

Snack: Sliced cucumber and carrot sticks with hummus.

Dinner: Baked salmon with a side of steamed broccoli and brown rice.

Achieving Optimal Health

The Type A diet isn't just about what to eat; it's about harnessing your blood type to achieve optimal health and vitality. By aligning your nutrition with your Type A status, you can enjoy improved digestion, increased energy, and a reduced risk of health issues.

Embrace your Type A status as a valuable piece of your unique health puzzle. By making informed dietary choices and embracing a lifestyle that aligns with your blood type, you can experience greater well-being and live your life to the fullest. Your journey to a healthier and more vibrant you starts here, with a deeper understanding of your genetic heritage and a commitment to nurturing your health and happiness.

Type B: The Nomads

In this chapter, we embark on an intriguing exploration of Type B individuals, often affectionately referred to as "The Nomads" among the blood types. If you're a Type B, you're about to uncover how your blood type can significantly influence your dietary preferences and health, providing you with a personalized roadmap to enhanced well-being.

Type B Characteristics

Type B individuals are thought to have emerged as a response to the globalization of human diets. As "The Nomads," they exhibit a set of distinctive characteristics that make them unique:

Adaptability: Type B individuals are known for their adaptability. They can comfortably accommodate a wide range of foods and environments.

Balanced Immune System: They typically possess a well-balanced immune system that can effectively fight off various infections.

Moderate Stomach Acid: Their stomach acid levels are moderate, allowing them to digest most foods without difficulty.

Prone to Autoimmune Conditions: Type B individuals may be more prone to certain autoimmune conditions. Therefore, it's essential to be mindful of their overall health and well-being.

The Type B Diet

The Type B diet is tailored to complement their genetic makeup, emphasizing foods that support their overall health and vitality. Here are key dietary recommendations for Type B individuals:

Varied Diet: Type B individuals should focus on a varied diet that includes a wide range of foods, including lean meats, fish, dairy, fruits, and vegetables.

Limit Certain Foods: While they can eat many foods with ease, they should reduce or eliminate specific items, such as corn, lentils, and sesame seeds.

Balanced Proteins: Type B individuals can enjoy a mix of animal proteins like poultry, fish, and lean meats, along with plant-based protein sources like legumes and nuts.

Dairy Products: Most Type B individuals can tolerate dairy products well. However, they should choose low-fat or fermented options for better health.

Moderation and Balance: To maintain their overall well-being, Type B individuals should practice moderation and balance in their diet and lifestyle.

Meal Planning for Type B

Creating balanced, satisfying meals for Type B individuals involves a mix of food groups and flavors. Here's an example of a Type B meal plan:

Breakfast: Greek yogurt with mixed berries and a sprinkle of almonds.

Lunch: Grilled chicken breast with a side of mixed greens and quinoa salad.

Snack: Hummus and vegetable sticks.

Dinner: Baked salmon with asparagus and a sweet potato.

Achieving Optimal Health

The Type B diet isn't merely about what to eat; it's about utilizing your blood type to attain the best possible health and well-being. By aligning your nutrition with your Type B status, you can experience enhanced digestion, increased energy levels, and a lower risk of health-related issues.

Embrace your Type B identity as a source of strength and adaptability, and recognize that your dietary choices can play a significant role in your overall vitality. Your journey to a healthier and more vibrant you begin here, with a deeper understanding of your genetic heritage and a commitment to nurturing your health and happiness.

Type AB: The Enigmas

Welcome to the intriguing world of Type AB individuals, often affectionately referred to as "The Enigmas" among the blood types. If you're a Type AB, get ready to embark on a journey of self-discovery as we explore how your blood type influences your dietary preferences and health, providing you with a personalized roadmap to enhanced well-being.

Type AB Characteristics

Type AB individuals are considered the newest blood type, a result of the intermingling of bloodlines and genetic diversity. As "The Enigmas," they exhibit a set of distinctive characteristics that make them unique:

Adaptability: Type AB individuals are known for their adaptability, blending traits of both Type A and Type B. They can comfortably accommodate a wide range of foods and environments.

Balanced Immune System: They typically possess a well-balanced immune system that can effectively fight off various infections.

Prone to Autoimmune Conditions: Like Type B individuals, Type AB individuals may be more prone to certain autoimmune conditions. It's crucial to be mindful of their overall health and well-being.

Complex Mix: Their blood type represents a unique combination of traits from Type A and Type B, making them a fascinating blend of characteristics.

The Type AB Diet

The Type AB diet is designed to complement their genetic makeup, emphasizing foods that support their overall health and vitality. Here are key dietary recommendations for Type AB individuals:

Balanced Diet: Type AB individuals should focus on a balanced diet that includes a variety of foods from both plant and animal sources. Lean meats, fish, dairy, fruits, and vegetables all have a place in their diet.

Avoid Certain Foods: While they can consume a wide range of foods, Type AB individuals should avoid items like processed meat, excessive red meat, and caffeine.

Proteins: They can enjoy a mix of animal proteins like poultry, fish, and lean meats, along with plant-based protein sources like tofu and legumes.

Dairy Products: Most Type AB individuals can tolerate dairy products well. Opt for low-fat or fermented options for better health.

Moderation and Balance: To maintain their overall well-being, Type AB individuals should practice moderation and balance in their diet and lifestyle.

Meal Planning for Type AB

Creating balanced, satisfying meals for Type AB individuals involves a harmonious blend of different foods. Here's an example of a Type AB meal plan:

Breakfast: Scrambled eggs with spinach and a side of mixed berries.

Lunch: Grilled chicken breast with a side of mixed greens and quinoa salad.

Snack: Greek yogurt with honey and almonds.

Dinner: Baked salmon with steamed asparagus and a sweet potato.

Achieving Optimal Health

The Type AB diet isn't just about what to eat; it's about leveraging your unique blood type to attain the best possible health and well-being. By aligning your nutrition with your Type AB identity, you can experience enhanced digestion, increased energy levels, and a lower risk of health-related issues.

Embrace your Type AB identity as a fascinating blend of characteristics, and recognize that your dietary choices can play a significant role in your overall vitality. Your journey to a healthier and more vibrant you starts here, with a deeper understanding of your genetic heritage and a commitment to nurturing your health and happiness.

Tailoring Nutrition to Your Blood Type

Your blood type isn't just a random label; it's a key to unlocking the door to personalized nutrition. In this chapter, we'll explore how you can tailor your diet to your specific blood type, Type O, Type A, Type B, or Type AB. By doing so, you can harness the power of your genetic makeup to optimize your health and well-being.

Understanding the Concept

The concept of tailoring nutrition to your blood type is rooted in the idea that our blood type influences the way our bodies react to different foods. Each blood type is associated with unique characteristics, vulnerabilities, and strengths, and this knowledge can be used to craft a diet that suits your individual needs.

Customized Nutrition for Each Blood Type

Let's dive into the specifics of how you can tailor your nutrition to your blood type:

Type O:
- Embrace a high-protein diet, including lean meats, fish, and poultry.

- Limit or avoid dairy and gluten-containing grains.
- Incorporate a balance of fruits and vegetables for fiber and antioxidants.
- Engage in regular, vigorous exercise for optimal results.

Type A:
- Thrive on a plant-based diet rich in vegetables, fruits, legumes, and whole grains.
- Reduce or eliminate animal proteins, particularly red meat.
- Be mindful of stress management and practice relaxation techniques.
- Engage in gentle, holistic exercises like yoga or tai chi.

Type B:
- Enjoy a balanced diet that includes a variety of foods from both plant and animal sources.
- Emphasize lean meats, fish, dairy, and plant-based proteins.
- Practice moderation and balance in your diet and lifestyle.
- Engage in diverse, enjoyable physical activities.

Type AB:

- Maintain a balanced diet, combining elements of both Type A and Type B recommendations.
- Enjoy a mix of animal proteins, including poultry, fish, and lean meats, along with plant-based protein sources.
- Be mindful of stress management and overall health.
- Practice moderation and balance in your diet and lifestyle.

Benefits of Tailored Nutrition

The advantages of aligning your diet with your blood type are numerous:

Enhanced Digestion: Eating foods that align with your blood type can lead to improved digestion and nutrient absorption.

Increased Energy: A tailored diet can provide you with more sustained energy throughout the day.

Reduced Health Risks: By addressing your genetic vulnerabilities, you can reduce the risk of certain health conditions.

Optimized Well-Being: Tailoring your nutrition to your blood type can lead to an overall sense of well-being and vitality.

Practical Application

Applying the principles of blood-type-based nutrition involves self-awareness and experimentation. Start by identifying your blood type through a reliable test, and then gradually modify your diet to align with the recommendations specific to your type.

Remember that while blood type-based nutrition offers a personalized approach, it's still important to maintain a balanced, overall diet and lifestyle. Individual factors, such as allergies and sensitivities, should also be considered.

Your journey to healthier and more vibrant living begins with understanding and appreciating your unique genetic heritage. By tailoring your nutrition to your blood type, you're taking a meaningful step towards a healthier, happier you.

Chapter 3

Exercise and Blood Type

Fitness Recommendations for Each Blood Type

Exercise is a vital component of a healthy lifestyle, but what works well for one person may not be as effective for another. In this chapter, we explore how your blood type can guide your fitness routine. Discover how to tailor your exercise regimen to your specific blood type, Type O, Type A, Type B, or Type AB, unlocking the potential for better fitness and overall well-being.

The Connection Between Blood Type and Exercise

Just as your blood type influences your dietary preferences, it also plays a role in determining the type of exercise that best suits your body. By understanding your blood type and its associated traits, you can select workouts that align with your unique needs and maximize your fitness goals.

Fitness Recommendations for Each Blood Type
Let's dive into the specific exercise recommendations for each blood type:

Type O:
High-Intensity Workouts: Type O individuals thrive on intense physical activity. Engage in activities like strength training, interval training, and cardio workouts.
Outdoor Activities: Spend time in the great outdoors, such as hiking, running, and obstacle courses.
Variation: Incorporate a variety of exercises to prevent boredom and challenge your body.

Type A:
Mind-Body Activities: Type A individuals benefit from mind-body exercises like yoga, tai chi, and Pilates.
Low-Impact Aerobics: Participate in low-impact aerobics or swimming to maintain cardiovascular health.
Consistency: Regular, gentle exercise routines that focus on flexibility and relaxation work best.

Type B:
Diverse Workouts: Type B individuals should incorporate a mix of different exercises, including cardio, strength training, and flexibility exercises.

Playful Activities: Engage in enjoyable physical activities such as dance, hiking, or martial arts.

Variation: Change up your workouts to keep things interesting and challenge your body.

Type AB:

Hybrid Workouts: Type AB individuals can benefit from a blend of mind-body activities like yoga and strength training.

Dance and Flexibility: Consider activities like dance or barre classes for an all-around fitness approach.

Moderation and Balance: Maintain a consistent fitness routine, but be mindful of not overexerting yourself.

Benefits of Blood Type-Appropriate Exercise

Aligning your fitness routine with your blood type offers numerous advantages:

Improved Results: Exercise routines tailored to your blood type can lead to better fitness outcomes.

Reduced Risk of Injury: Choosing the right exercises for your body type can lower the risk of injury.

Enhanced Well-Being: Blood type-appropriate workouts can improve your overall sense of well-being.

Practical Application

To apply blood type-based fitness recommendations, start by identifying your blood type. Then, experiment with different exercises and observe how your body responds. Pay attention to your energy levels, muscle soreness, and overall satisfaction with the workout.

Remember that individual factors, such as age, fitness level, and any pre-existing health conditions, should also be considered when designing your exercise routine. The key is to find a fitness regimen that not only suits your blood type but also suits you as a unique individual.

Your fitness journey is about more than just following the latest trends. It's about understanding and respecting your body's inherent traits and choosing exercises that empower you to become the healthiest and happiest version of yourself. By aligning your exercise routine with your blood type, you're taking a step toward a fitter, more vibrant you.

Customizing Workout Routines

In the world of fitness, one size does not fit all. Customizing your workout routine to align with your individual needs, goals, and abilities is a cornerstone of successful and sustainable fitness. In this chapter, we explore the art of tailoring your exercise regimen to suit you, regardless of your blood type.

The Importance of Customization

No two people are identical, and what works for one person may not be effective or enjoyable for another. This is why customizing your workout routine is vital for achieving your fitness objectives while maintaining motivation and ensuring long-term success. Here's why it's so important:

Optimal Results: Tailoring your workouts ensures that you're targeting the right muscle groups and energy systems to achieve the results you desire.

Injury Prevention: Customized routines help you avoid overexertion and the risk of injury by working within your physical limits.

Sustainability: When your workouts are enjoyable and suited to your preferences, you're more likely to stick with them in the long run.

Variety and Fun: Customization allows you to incorporate a variety of exercises and activities that you genuinely enjoy.

Designing Your Customized Workout

Creating a customized workout routine involves several key steps:

1. Set Clear Goals

Define your fitness objectives, whether it's weight loss, muscle gain, increased flexibility, or enhanced endurance.

2. Assess Your Current Fitness Level

Understand where you are in terms of strength, flexibility, and cardiovascular fitness. This forms the foundation for your customized plan.

3. Choose Activities You Enjoy

Find exercises and activities that you genuinely like. This ensures that your workouts are something you look forward to, rather than something you dread.

4. Incorporate Variety

Include a mix of exercises to target different muscle groups and energy systems. This keeps your workouts interesting and challenges your body in various ways.

5. Create a Balanced Routine

Ensure that your routine covers all essential components of fitness, including cardiovascular exercise, strength training, flexibility, and balance work.

6. Adjust Intensity and Duration

Tailor the intensity and duration of your workouts based on your fitness level and goals. Gradually progress as you become more fit.

7. Listen to Your Body

Pay attention to how your body responds to exercise. Adapt your routine as needed to accommodate any physical limitations, soreness, or other factors.

8. Seek Professional Guidance

If you're new to exercise or have specific health concerns, consider consulting a fitness professional or healthcare provider to help you create a safe and effective customized workout.

The Role of Blood Type

While blood type can provide some guidance for exercise recommendations, it should not be the sole determinant of your workout routine. Your personal preferences, fitness goals, and body's response to exercise should be the primary factors driving your choices. The goal is to use your blood type-based knowledge as one of many tools to enhance your fitness journey.

Conclusion

Customizing your workout routine is an empowering way to achieve your fitness goals while ensuring that exercise remains an enjoyable and sustainable part of your life. By taking the time to assess your needs, set clear objectives, and listen to your body, you can design a personalized exercise plan that leads to improved health, well-being, and fitness. Your journey to a fitter, healthier, and happier you begin with the understanding that your workouts should be as unique as you are.

Chapter 4

Mind-Body Connection

Psychological and Emotional Aspects Linked to Blood Types

Your blood type is not only a biological classification; it can also offer insights into the psychological and emotional aspects that shape your personality, reactions, and behaviors. In this chapter, we explore the intriguing links between blood types and the mind-body connection, helping you gain a deeper understanding of how your blood type can influence your psychological and emotional well-being.

The Complex Interplay

The connection between blood type and personality or emotional traits is a complex and evolving field of study. While it's essential to recognize that blood type is just one of many factors that shape an individual, it can provide valuable insights into certain tendencies and predispositions. Here are some key associations:

Type O:

Proactive and Strong-Willed: Type O individuals are often described as assertive, outgoing, and goal-oriented.

Optimistic: They tend to have a positive outlook and may handle stress well.

Impulsive: They may be more prone to spontaneous decision-making.

Type A:

Sensitive and Considerate: Type A individuals are often seen as thoughtful, compassionate, and detail-oriented.

Stress-Prone: They might be more susceptible to stress and anxiety.

Introverted: Type A individuals may lean toward introversion, seeking solace in quieter, reflective activities.

Type B:

Flexible and Creative: Type B individuals are often recognized for their adaptability, creativity, and open-mindedness.

Prone to Indecision: They may struggle with decision-making due to their desire to consider multiple perspectives.

Relaxed Approach: Type B individuals generally approach life with a more relaxed and laid-back attitude.

Type AB:

Adaptable and Complex Thinkers: Type AB individuals possess the ability to understand complex concepts and adapt to various situations.

Dual Nature: They may exhibit a duality in their personality, combining traits from both Type A and Type B.

Creative and Sensitive: Type AB individuals often excel in artistic and empathetic endeavors.

Embracing the Mind-Body Connection

Understanding the psychological and emotional aspects linked to your blood type is not about being confined to a particular set of traits. It's about recognizing tendencies and using this knowledge to promote self-awareness and personal growth. Here's how to embrace the mind-body connection:

Self-Reflection: Take time to reflect on your unique qualities, strengths, and areas where you may want to grow.

Embrace Diversity: Recognize that blood type is just one piece of the puzzle. People with the same blood type can have very different personalities.

Stress Management: If your blood type is associated with stress susceptibility, focus on stress management techniques that work for you, such as mindfulness, exercise, or social support.

Self-Care: Tailor your self-care routines, including hobbies and activities, to suit your personality and emotional well-being.

Personal Growth: Use your knowledge of your tendencies to set goals for personal development and work on areas you want to improve.

Conclusion

The mind-body connection, influenced by your blood type, is a fascinating aspect of human diversity. Recognizing how your blood type may relate to your personality and emotional tendencies can be a valuable tool for self-discovery and personal growth. Embrace your individuality, harness your strengths, and work on areas that may require attention to create a more fulfilled and balanced you. Your journey towards greater self-awareness and well-being starts with understanding the connection between your blood type and your mind and emotions.

Stress Management Techniques

In today's fast-paced world, stress has become a common companion in many lives. Managing stress is essential for maintaining overall well-being. Here are various techniques that can help you effectively cope with and reduce stress.

Mindfulness and Meditation

Mindfulness Practice: Engage in mindfulness activities that bring your focus to the present moment. This could include mindful breathing, observing your surroundings, or practicing gratitude.

Meditation: Dedicate time to meditation, allowing yourself to find a quiet space, focus on your breath, and let go of racing thoughts. Guided meditations or meditation apps can be helpful for beginners.

Physical Activity and Exercise

Regular Exercise: Engage in physical activities that you enjoy, whether it's going for a walk, hitting the gym, dancing, or practicing yoga. Exercise releases endorphins, which are natural stress fighters.

Yoga and Tai Chi: These mind-body practices not only improve physical flexibility but also promote mental calmness and relaxation.

Breathing and Relaxation Techniques

Deep Breathing: Take slow, deep breaths, focusing on the rhythm of your breathing. This technique can be done anywhere and helps calm your nervous system.

Progressive Muscle Relaxation: This involves tensing and relaxing each muscle group in your body. It's a systematic way to release tension and induce relaxation.

Time Management and Organization

Prioritize Tasks: Break tasks into smaller, manageable parts and prioritize them to avoid feeling overwhelmed.

Use a Planner or Calendar: Organize your day or week, setting specific times for work, relaxation, and personal activities. This can provide a sense of control over your schedule.

Social Support and Connection

Talk to Someone: Reach out to friends, family, or a professional for support and guidance. Sometimes, just talking about your stress can relieve some of the pressure.

Maintain Relationships: Nurturing healthy relationships can provide emotional support and a sense of belonging, reducing stress levels.

Hobbies and Relaxation Techniques

Engage in Hobbies: Dedicate time to activities you enjoy, whether it's painting, reading, gardening, or playing an instrument. These activities can act as a form of stress relief.

Take Breaks: Give yourself regular breaks from work or stressful situations. Even a short walk or a few moments of deep breathing can make a significant difference.

Healthy Lifestyle Habits

Balanced Diet: Eating a nutritious diet can positively impact your stress levels. Avoid excessive caffeine and sugar, and focus on consuming balanced, whole foods.

Adequate Sleep: Ensure you're getting enough quality sleep. Lack of sleep can significantly increase stress levels.

Conclusion

Managing stress involves finding what works best for you. Experiment with various techniques and combinations to discover what helps you relax and unwind. It's important to note that stress management is a continuous process, and what works during one period of your life might need adjustments in another. Prioritize your well-being and explore these techniques to find what aids you in managing stress effectively in your unique circumstances.

Chapter 5

Blood Type and Disease Prevention

Disease Susceptibility Based on Blood Type

The relationship between blood type and disease susceptibility is a subject of ongoing research and fascination. In this chapter, we delve into the intriguing connections between blood type and certain health conditions. Understanding how your blood type may influence disease susceptibility can empower you to make informed decisions about your health and well-being.

The Blood Type and Disease Link

While the exact mechanisms aren't fully understood, researchers have uncovered correlations between blood type and certain diseases. These associations offer valuable insights into potential risks and preventive measures. Here's a look at some of the key links:

Blood Type O:

Lower Risk of Heart Disease: Type O individuals tend to have a lower risk of heart disease and stroke.

Higher Risk of Ulcers: They may be more susceptible to peptic ulcers, which are sores in the stomach or small intestine.

Lower Risk of Blood Clots: Type O individuals might have a decreased risk of blood clot formation.

Blood Type A:

Increased Risk of Heart Disease: Type A individuals may have a higher risk of heart disease and hypertension.

Higher Cancer Risk: They might be more prone to certain cancers, such as stomach and breast cancer.

Lower Risk of Blood Clots: Type A individuals tend to have a decreased risk of blood clot formation.

Blood Type B:

Lower Risk of Heart Disease: Type B individuals may have a lower risk of heart disease compared to other blood types.

Increased Risk of Autoimmune Diseases: They may be more susceptible to certain autoimmune conditions, like lupus and multiple sclerosis.

Blood Type AB:
Increased Risk of Cognitive Decline: Type AB individuals might be at a higher risk of cognitive decline in older age.

Higher Cancer Risk: They may be more susceptible to certain cancers, such as stomach and ovarian cancer.

Disease Prevention and Management

While your blood type may influence disease susceptibility, it's essential to remember that genetics is just one piece of the puzzle. Lifestyle factors, such as diet, exercise, and stress management, play significant roles in disease prevention and management. Here's how you can use this knowledge to your advantage:

Tailored Nutrition: Consider adopting a diet that aligns with your blood type to address potential vulnerabilities and reduce associated risks.

Physical Activity: Engage in regular exercise to maintain cardiovascular health, strengthen your immune system, and reduce the risk of various diseases.

Stress Management: Implement stress management techniques to mitigate potential stress-related risks.

Regular Check-ups: Regardless of your blood type, regular health check-ups are crucial for early detection and prevention of diseases.

Individualized Care: If you have a family history of certain diseases, discuss your risk factors with a healthcare professional to create a personalized prevention plan.

Conclusion

Your blood type can provide insights into potential health risks, but it's only part of the story. It's vital to remember that genetics is not destiny, and you have the power to make choices that positively impact your health. By understanding the links between blood type and disease susceptibility, you can take proactive steps to minimize risks and maximize your overall well-being. Your journey to a healthier, disease-free future begins with knowledge, awareness, and a commitment to a healthy lifestyle.

Strategies for Disease Prevention

Preventing disease and maintaining good health is a lifelong endeavor that involves a combination of healthy lifestyle choices, regular medical check-ups, and risk reduction. By implementing effective disease prevention strategies, you can significantly lower your risk of developing various health conditions. Here are some key strategies to help you on your path to disease prevention:

1. Maintain a Balanced Diet

A well-balanced diet is a cornerstone of disease prevention. Follow these dietary guidelines to help protect your health:

Eat a Variety of Foods: Consume a wide range of fruits, vegetables, whole grains, lean proteins, and healthy fats to ensure you get a variety of essential nutrients.

Limit Sugar and Processed Foods: Reduce your intake of sugary beverages, processed snacks, and high-sugar foods, as they are linked to obesity and chronic diseases.

Control Portion Sizes: Be mindful of portion sizes to avoid overeating, which can lead to weight gain and related health issues.

Stay Hydrated: Drink plenty of water and limit sugary drinks and excessive caffeine.

2. Regular Physical Activity

Exercise is not only essential for maintaining a healthy weight but also for promoting overall well-being. Incorporate physical activity into your daily routine with the following tips:

Aim for Regular Exercise: Strive for at least 150 minutes of moderate-intensity aerobic exercise or 75 minutes of vigorous-intensity aerobic exercise per week, along with muscle-strengthening activities.

Find Activities You Enjoy: Engage in physical activities you love, whether it's hiking, dancing, swimming, or playing sports. This makes exercise more enjoyable and sustainable.

Stay Consistent: Make exercise a regular part of your life to reap the long-term benefits.

3. Stress Management

Chronic stress can have a detrimental impact on your health. Implement stress management techniques to reduce its negative effects:

Practice Relaxation Techniques: Engage in practices like meditation, deep breathing, and yoga to reduce stress and improve overall well-being.

Maintain Work-Life Balance: Strive for a healthy balance between work, family, and personal time.

Seek Support: Don't hesitate to seek support from friends, family, or a mental health professional if you're dealing with chronic stress.

4. Regular Health Check-ups

Regular medical check-ups are crucial for early detection and prevention of diseases. Consult with your healthcare provider to establish a schedule that includes:

Annual Physical Exams: These exams can help detect health issues early.

Screenings: Follow recommended screening guidelines for conditions like cancer, heart disease, and diabetes.

Immunizations: Stay up-to-date with vaccinations to prevent infectious diseases.

5. Tobacco and Alcohol Control

Tobacco and excessive alcohol consumption are major risk factors for many diseases. Consider these steps:

Quit Smoking: If you smoke, seek support to quit, as it's one of the most significant steps you can take for your health.

Moderate Alcohol Consumption: Limit alcohol to moderate levels, which is typically defined as one drink per day for women and up to two drinks per day for men.

6. Disease-Specific Prevention

Some diseases have unique prevention strategies. Be aware of your risk factors and take appropriate actions:

Heart Disease: Maintain a heart-healthy diet, control blood pressure and cholesterol, and engage in regular exercise.

Cancer: Follow screening recommendations, such as mammograms and colonoscopies, and reduce exposure to risk factors like smoking and excessive sun exposure.

Diabetes: Monitor blood sugar levels, maintain a healthy weight and engage in regular physical activity.

Conclusion

Disease prevention is a proactive approach to health that involves making informed lifestyle choices and staying up-to-date with medical recommendations. By adopting a well-balanced diet, staying physically active, managing stress, and being proactive about your health, you can significantly reduce your risk of developing various diseases. Remember that disease prevention is an ongoing commitment, and small, consistent steps can lead to significant improvements in your overall health and well-being.

By implementing effective disease prevention strategies, you can significantly lower your risk of developing various health conditions.

Chapter 6

Meal Plans and Recipes

Sample Meal Plans for Each Blood Type

One of the practical ways to align your nutrition with your blood type is by creating meal plans that cater to your specific dietary needs. In this chapter, we provide sample meal plans for each blood type.Type O, Type A, Type B, and Type AB. These meal plans offer a starting point for tailoring your diet to optimize your health and well-being.

Type O Meal Plan
Breakfast:

- Scrambled eggs with spinach and sliced tomato
- Fresh fruit salad with berries and melon

Lunch:

- Grilled chicken breast on a mixed greens salad
- Steamed broccoli and carrots

Snack:

- Greek yogurt with honey and walnuts

Dinner:

- Baked salmon with asparagus
- Quinoa cooked with a side of sautéed spinach

Type A Meal Plan

Breakfast:

- Oatmeal topped with sliced bananas and almonds
- Green tea

Lunch:

- Lentil soup with a side salad of mixed greens
- Fresh fruit

Snack:

- Hummus with vegetable sticks

Dinner:

- Grilled tofu with steamed broccoli and brown rice
- Herbal tea

Type B Meal Plan

Breakfast:

- Greek yogurt with honey and mixed berries
- Whole-grain toast with almond butter

Lunch:
- Turkey and avocado sandwich on whole-grain bread
- Mixed greens salad

Snack:
- Sliced apples with peanut butter

Dinner:
- Stir-fried shrimp with a variety of colorful vegetables
- Jasmine rice

Type AB Meal Plan
Breakfast:
- Scrambled eggs with sautéed mushrooms and a slice of whole-grain toast
- Fresh orange juice

Lunch:
- Quinoa salad with grilled chicken and mixed vegetables
- Fresh fruit salad

Snack:

- Greek yogurt with sliced almonds

Dinner:

- Baked fish with a side of roasted sweet potatoes and green beans
- Chamomile tea

Tips for Customizing Meal Plans

While these meal plans are tailored to each blood type, they are not set in stone. You can customize them to suit your preferences and dietary needs. Here are some general guidelines for customization:

Portion Control: Adjust portion sizes to align with your calorie requirements and appetite.

Food Variations: Within your blood type's recommendations, experiment with different foods and flavors to keep your meals interesting.

Allergies and Sensitivities: Take into account any food allergies or sensitivities you have when customizing your meals.

Nutrient Balance: Ensure your meals provide a balance of macronutrients (carbohydrates, proteins, and fats) and include a variety of nutrients.

Hydration: Don't forget to stay well-hydrated by consuming an adequate amount of water or other healthy beverages throughout the day.

Desserts and Treats: While it's important to focus on nutritious foods, don't forget to include occasional treats in your meal plans to satisfy cravings and maintain a balanced approach to eating.

Conclusion

Creating meal plans that align with your blood type can be a practical way to optimize your diet and overall health. Use the sample meal plans provided for each blood type as a starting point, and then tailor them to your specific tastes, dietary needs, and preferences. Remember that your journey to better health and well-being begins with a deeper understanding of your genetic heritage and a commitment to nurturing your health and happiness through a personalized approach to nutrition.

Delicious Recipes Tailored to Specific Blood Types

Type O: Grilled Chicken and Vegetable Skewers

Ingredients:

- 2 boneless, skinless chicken breasts, cut into chunks
- Bell peppers (red, yellow, and green), cut into chunks
- Red onion, cut into chunks
- Zucchini, sliced
- Cherry tomatoes
- Olive oil
- Garlic powder
- Oregano
- Salt and pepper
- Wooden skewers, soaked in water

Instructions:

1. In a bowl, mix olive oil, garlic powder, oregano, salt, and pepper to create a marinade.

2. Thread chicken, bell peppers, red onion, zucchini, and cherry tomatoes onto the skewers.

3. Brush the skewers with the marinade.

4. Preheat your grill to medium-high heat.

5. Grill the skewers for about 10-12 minutes, turning occasionally, until the chicken is cooked through.

6. Serve with a side of quinoa or a fresh green salad.

Type A: Lentil and Vegetable Soup

Ingredients:
- 1 cup green or brown lentils
- 1 onion, chopped
- 2 carrots, sliced
- 2 celery stalks, chopped
- 1 zucchini, diced
- 1 can of diced tomatoes
- 4 cups vegetable broth
- 2 cloves garlic, minced
- Thyme
- Bay leaves
- Salt and pepper
- Olive oil

Instructions:
1. In a large pot, heat olive oil and sauté the chopped onion, garlic, carrots, and celery until they start to soften.
2. Add lentils, zucchini, diced tomatoes, thyme, and bay leaves.

3. Pour in the vegetable broth and bring to a boil.

4. Reduce heat, cover, and simmer for about 25-30 minutes, or until the lentils and vegetables are tender.

5. Season with salt and pepper to taste.

6. Serve hot with a side of whole-grain bread.

Type B: Grilled Salmon with Lemon-Dill Sauce

Ingredients:

- 2 salmon fillets
- Lemon juice
- Fresh dill, chopped
- Olive oil
- Garlic, minced
- Salt and pepper

Instructions:

1. In a bowl, mix olive oil, lemon juice, fresh dill, minced garlic, salt, and pepper to create a marinade.

2. Brush the marinade over the salmon fillets and let them marinate for about 15-30 minutes.

3. Preheat your grill to medium-high heat.

4. Grill the salmon for about 4-5 minutes per side or until it flakes easily with a fork.

5. Serve with a side of steamed asparagus and brown rice.

Type AB: Vegetable Stir-Fry with Tofu

Ingredients:
- 1 block of tofu, cubed
- Mixed vegetables (broccoli, bell peppers, snap peas, carrots)
- Low-sodium soy sauce or tamari
- Fresh ginger, grated
- Garlic, minced
- Sesame oil
- Brown rice

Instructions:

1. In a pan, heat sesame oil and sauté tofu until it's golden brown. Remove and set aside.

2. In the same pan, add more sesame oil and stir-fry the mixed vegetables until they're tender-crisp.

3. Add grated ginger and minced garlic to the vegetables.

4. Return the tofu to the pan and mix everything.

5. Drizzle with low-sodium soy sauce or tamari and stir to coat.

6. Serve over cooked brown rice.

These recipes are a starting point for tailoring your meals to your specific blood type. Customize them further by adding or omitting ingredients according to your tastes and preferences. Enjoy your delicious, blood type-appropriate meals!

Chapter 7

Fine-Tuning Your Lifestyle

Implementing Blood Type Strategies in Daily Life

As you've delved into the world of blood type-based nutrition and lifestyle recommendations, you've gained valuable insights into how your unique blood type can influence your health and well-being. Now, it's time to fine-tune your lifestyle to align with these strategies. In this chapter, we explore practical ways to implement blood type recommendations in your daily life.

Blood Type and Your Daily Routine

Understanding the connections between your blood type and various aspects of your life, including diet, exercise, and stress management, empowers you to make more informed choices. Here are some steps to integrate blood type strategies into your daily routine:

1. Meal Planning and Grocery Shopping

Create Blood Type-Friendly Menus: Use the sample meal plans provided earlier and customize them to suit your tastes. Plan your meals to ensure you have the right ingredients on hand.

Read Food Labels: When grocery shopping, carefully read food labels to make informed choices about the products you buy. Look for foods that align with your blood type recommendations.

Stock Up on Staples: Keep blood-type-appropriate staples in your pantry and fridge so that you always have the basis for a healthy meal.

2. Fitness and Exercise

Choose Suitable Workouts: Tailor your exercise routine to match your blood type's recommendations. If you're Type O, opt for high-intensity workouts, while Type A individuals may focus on mind-body activities.

Consistency Matters: Make exercise a consistent part of your routine to reap the long-term benefits. Find activities you genuinely enjoy to keep your motivation high.

Listen to Your Body: Pay attention to how your body responds to exercise. Adjust your routine as needed to accommodate any physical limitations or fluctuations in your health.

3. Stress Management

Practice Stress Reduction Techniques: Incorporate stress management techniques into your daily life. This could be as simple as a morning meditation or regular deep-breathing exercises.

Set Boundaries: Establish clear boundaries to maintain a healthy work-life balance. Avoid overcommitting or overextending yourself.

Seek Support: Don't hesitate to reach out to friends, family, or professionals when stress becomes overwhelming. Share your challenges and seek advice or support.

4. Health Check-ups

Regular Health Check-ups: Schedule regular check-ups with your healthcare provider. Share your blood type knowledge and discuss how it may relate to your health and specific risks.

Screening and Prevention: Follow recommended screening guidelines for your age and gender, and work with your healthcare provider to address specific disease prevention strategies that align with your blood type.

5. Individualized Approach

Remember that while your blood type provides useful insights, it's just one of many factors that influence your health. Individual variations, such as age, genetics, and personal preferences, also play significant roles. Here are some additional tips for fine-tuning your lifestyle:

Flexibility: Be flexible and open to adaptation. If you find a particular strategy isn't working for you, don't hesitate to make changes.

Self-Reflection: Continuously assess your well-being and how the strategies are working for you. Adjust as needed to optimize your health and happiness.

Seek Professional Guidance: If you're unsure about how to fine-tune your lifestyle according to your blood type, consult with a healthcare provider, nutritionist, or fitness professional for expert advice and support.

Conclusion

Fine-tuning your lifestyle to align with your blood type strategies is a journey of self-discovery and self-improvement. By implementing these recommendations into your daily life, you can harness the power of personalized health and well-being. Remember that it's not about rigidly adhering to a set of rules but about using your blood type knowledge as a valuable tool to lead a happier, healthier, and more fulfilling life. Your journey towards better living is an ongoing adventure that starts with the understanding that you have the power to make informed choices and take charge of your well-being.

Overcoming Challenges and Adapting to Individual Needs

In your journey to implement blood-type-based strategies in your life, you may encounter various challenges and obstacles that require adaptation and resilience. Understanding how to overcome these challenges and make necessary adjustments is a vital aspect of optimizing your health and well-being. Here, we'll explore common challenges and guide how to adapt to your individual needs.

Challenge 1: Social and Cultural Pressures

Adaptation: When faced with social and cultural pressures that conflict with your blood type-based choices, it's essential to find a balance that suits you. Here's how:

Effective Communication: Communicate your choices politely but assertively to those who may question your dietary or lifestyle decisions.

Plan Ahead: When attending social gatherings or dining out, plan by researching menu options that align with your blood type. You can also eat beforehand or bring your dish.

Educate Others: Share information about blood type-based strategies with friends and family, helping them understand your choices better.

Challenge 2: Cravings and Taste Preferences

Adaptation: Managing cravings and taste preferences can be challenging, but it's not insurmountable. Here's how to navigate this obstacle:

Gradual Changes: Make gradual dietary changes to allow your taste buds to adjust to new flavors and preferences.

Seek Alternatives: Find blood type-compliant alternatives that satisfy your cravings. For example, if you crave sweets, consider natural sweeteners like honey or maple syrup.

Variety and Creativity: Experiment with a variety of foods and cooking techniques to keep your meals interesting and flavorful.

Challenge 3: Lifestyle Constraints

Adaptation: Balancing blood type-based strategies with the demands of your lifestyle can be challenging. Here's how to make the necessary adjustments:

Prioritize: Identify your health goals and prioritize them within your lifestyle constraints. This might involve allocating specific time for exercise or planning meals.

Incorporate Short Workouts: If you have a busy schedule, break down your exercise routine into short, effective workouts that can be done throughout the day.

Meal Prep: Spend time on meal planning and preparation to ensure that blood-type-compliant meals are readily available, even on the busiest days.

Challenge 4: Health Conditions

Adaptation: Individuals with pre-existing health conditions may face additional challenges in implementing blood type-based strategies. Here's how to adapt to your individual needs:

Consult a Healthcare Provider: If you have a medical condition, consult with a healthcare provider to discuss how blood type-based recommendations align with your specific health needs.

Medication Considerations: If you're on medication, ensure that your dietary choices do not interfere with your prescriptions. Discuss any potential conflicts with your healthcare provider.

Flexibility and Modification: Adapt your blood type-based strategies to accommodate your health condition. There may be specific recommendations that need modification based on your health.

Challenge 5: Sustainability

Adaptation: Maintaining a blood-type-based lifestyle in the long term can sometimes be challenging due to its sustainability. Here's how to make it a lasting part of your life:

Consistency: Consistency is key. Stay committed to your chosen path and view it as a long-term investment in your health.

Variety: Continually explore new recipes and foods within the framework of your blood type to keep your diet interesting.

Self-Care: Ensure you're taking care of your mental and emotional well-being, as this is essential for long-term lifestyle adherence.

Conclusion

Overcoming challenges and adapting to individual needs is an integral part of successfully implementing blood type-based strategies in your life. Remember that these strategies are meant to empower you, not restrict you. Embrace your uniqueness, be flexible, and make choices that align with your health and happiness. Your journey to optimized well-being is an ongoing process, and your ability to adapt and overcome challenges will play a significant role in your ultimate success.

Conclusion

Your journey through the world of blood type-based nutrition and lifestyle strategies has provided you with valuable insights into how to optimize your health and well-being. By understanding the connections between your blood type and various aspects of your life, you've gained the tools to make informed choices that can positively impact your overall health.

As you move forward, keep in mind that these strategies are not about rigid rules but rather about using your blood type knowledge as a valuable tool to lead a happier, healthier, and more fulfilling life. Here are some key takeaways from your journey:

1. Personalized Approach: Your blood type is just one piece of the puzzle, but it can help you create a more personalized approach to nutrition, exercise, stress management, and overall well-being.

2. Balanced Flexibility: While adhering to blood type recommendations, it's important to maintain a balanced sense of flexibility. Adaptation and customization are key to long-term success.

3. Self-Discovery: Your journey has been a path of self-discovery, allowing you to better understand your body, preferences, and how to nurture your health.

4. Resilience: Challenges and obstacles are a part of life, but your newfound knowledge empowers you to overcome them with resilience and adaptability.

5. Consistency: Consistency in implementing these strategies is the key to long-term health benefits. Stay committed to your chosen path.

6. Well-Being: Remember that your ultimate goal is well-being, happiness, and a life filled with vitality and joy. Blood type-based strategies are tools to help you achieve these goals.

Your journey doesn't end here. It continues as you fine-tune your lifestyle, adapt to individual needs, and embrace the power of personalized health. With the knowledge you've gained, you're equipped to make choices that promote a healthier, happier, and more fulfilling life. Your path to optimized well-being is ongoing, and it's a journey worth embracing with enthusiasm and dedication.